How to lose weight and get fit by Walking!

All the secrets of losing weight... walking

Andy Bakas

Acknowledgments

I would like to thank my teacher and mentor John Papadrak for the opportunity he gave me to change my life. He accompanied me on my own journey and was willing to transfer his wealth of knowledge and to help me to achieve my goals.

I would also like to thank all of our students and friends who have taught me so many useful things and made me a better person.

Our parents provide us with the care and support we need to progress along life's path. I sincerely thank mine for their never-ending belief and encouragement.

Introduction

Today's fast-paced lifestyles, packed with daily worries and problems cause all of us anxiety, stress and uncertainty. Many hours spent at work and little time to play mean we often end up forgoing any form of physical activity. The result is that many people neglect their health, resulting in weight gain and lack of vitality—and as time goes on, the emergence of health problems.

We frequently hear people saying they want to get fit and lose a little or a lot of weight. They are then faced with the dilemma of choosing the best way to lose weight, deciding which are the best diets out there, and then making sure they stick to a diet and overcome all the temptation so readily available these days.

In this book I will show you the best way to go about this and will reveal the secrets to achieving your target of weight loss, health, vitality and energy in your daily life.

Several years ago, I met my mentor and teacher John Papadrak. He was a professor at the university at which I was studying for my second degree. He was aged around fifty-five but looked much younger. He was an excellent mentor—tireless and bursting with incredible energy. I would often bump into him early in the morning as he walked at the university, complete with backpack and sports shoes—not your typical university professor. I was interested.

Some time later, we met in the framework of the course he taught and I started chatting to him about walking. That was when it all started.

John explained to me that he had suffered from health problems a few years back. His doctor had recommended that he lose a significant amount of weight as quickly as possible. He lived in London at the time, where he taught at a university. He tried to reduce the quantities of food he consumed, but although initially he lost some weight, he subsequently put it on back and ended up feeling miserable and disappointed.

Then he met someone who taught him the secrets of walking for weight loss. The idea of walking to lose weight sounded simple and appealing, and he decided to give it a try. Three months later, he had lost twenty kilos of fat (forty-four lbs) without any crash diets and without the feeling that he was trying to lose weight.

"The best way to reduce your food intake, do some sport and lose weight without feeling you are depriving yourself of anything is through walking," he used to tell me. Walking burns fat! Two to three weeks after you start walking at the pace described in the next chapters, you will really feel that you are burning fat from your body!

"What about running, swimming or other sports—don't they burn fat and help with weight loss?" I asked John.

"All physical activity promotes weight loss, but walking burns fat directly. Intense walking, the type that makes you puff and sweat, burns fat, while running directly transforms fat into muscle, unless you run a very long distance, which is rather difficult for a beginner with excess weight and bad eating habits. The big secret is that when we walk, our heart rate remains within 100 to 130 beats per minute, and it is at these rates that our body burns fat most effectively and directly."

I was already impressed by what I was hearing and felt I definitely wanted to give it a try. I had been jogging for a long time but didn't seem to be able to shift the excess kilos.

A few days later, I visited him in his office and asked him to show me how to walk and to teach me the secrets of weight loss and healthy living. He told me that his house was located eight kilometers (about five miles) away from the university. He used to walk from his home to the university each morning and back home each night. He suggested I follow him, on the condition that what I was about to learn from him I would teach to others, as he had done with me. I had no reason not to accept this condition; indeed there is nothing more rewarding than teaching other people the secrets of how to remain healthy, lose weight and feel energized.

Within thirty days, I had lost weight, gained vitality and just felt really wonderful. "Now the time has come to learn the secrets of the technique of walking as well as the right diet," John told me, and began to enumerate the secrets and tips that I am going to present, as succinctly as I can, in the following chapters.

My motivation to write this book is a desire to transfer this knowledge to as many people as possible, so that they, too, see how easy it is to lose weight through walking—and how easy and enjoyable walking is.
Most of us—myself included—can't even begin to imagine just how easy it is to lose weight through walking, and that replacing bad habits with good ones will have a global effect on our approach towards life. With all my heart, I suggest you try it.

Why not? After all, it's just... walking!

Chapter 1: Why Walking?

We are all keen to discover the activity or sport that will give us the best weight-loss results. The truth is that any physical activity helps to reduce weight. But there are significant differences from activity to activity. Why is walking considered one of the better, safer and healthier methods of reducing weight?

For more than twenty years I have personally tried almost all modes of fitness, running, swimming, cycling, team sports and body building. After a great deal of physical activity and a lot of thought, I discovered that walking is the ideal exercise for awakening a dormant metabolism. Many nutritionists recommend to their customers that they include walking in their everyday routine, to boost their metabolism.

The secret is that intense walking raises the pulse to between 100 and 130, the ideal rate to stimulate the body to eat stored fat. More intense exercise such as fast running converts fat into lean muscle mass. It is a known fact that many people who routinely run often do not observe a significant reduction in their weight, precisely because this form of exercise does not burn fat, but converts it into muscle mass.

Some facts about walking:

1. **Walking at the right pace, as described in the next chapter, brings the best results. It burns fat!**

2. It is extremely easy for someone to work out while walking. Walking can be made part of our everyday routine—the journey to and from work, weekend strolls or a walk with the family on a beautiful afternoon.

3. It is safe for our body and does not cause hidden damage such as that often caused to the knees by jogging or cycling. All you need is a pair of good shoes and your good mood!

4. It is the only exercise that can combine fitness and spirituality. Let me explain immediately what I mean. When someone is walking, they are easily able to focus on the activity at hand as well as listen to a smartphone, iPod or similar device containing their favorite

music audio book, courses, lectures and seminars. Walking enables us to focus our attention wholly on what we are listening to—something that is not possible when, for example, running or cycling because it's very hard to focus your attention mentally on listening. This is the reason athletes in these sports usually only listen to music while exercising. As I will describe below, this is an excellent form of self-motivation, especially for walking, for those who find it difficult to make exercise part of their daily routine.

5. It is easy to walk with friends and to enjoy a chat at the same time—something that is difficult, if not impossible, when running, cycling or swimming.

6. The instant results one sees in terms of health are fast and impressive. Almost from the first month, you will feel well and healthy, lucid and elegant.

7. The more you walk, the more you want. This is one of the incredible phenomena of walking. Because you are not pushing your body to its limits, it does not create negative associations in the brain, so slowly our brains become programmed to the fact that this activity is not troublesome and stress-inducing but instead gives us joy and euphoria.

8. It is ideal for people with a lot of excess weight. Most people who participate in my seminars and who start out significantly overweight continue to walk and stick to their exercise routine once they reach their goal and have shed many kilos. This in itself says a lot. My friend John K. weighed 120 kg (264 lbs); after eight months of daily walking and a sensible diet, he lost 40 kilos (88 lbs). Today he is slim and fit, still walking to and from work, and says that the best challenge for him is the numerous stairs at the university, which he always takes rather than the elevator…

9. Walking can be done anywhere, anytime and under any weather conditions. Whether it's raining cats and dogs, blowing gale-force winds or snowing, your daily walking exercise routine can go ahead—obviously with suitable clothing.

10. It is very good exercise, tightens the muscles of the legs and waist.

11. It stops hunger and cuts appetite. Generally speaking, most forms of physical activity reduce the sensation of hunger. This is particularly so in the case of intensive walking, which raises the heart rate to 100 to 130 beats per minute, creating an incredible sensation of satiety that slowly makes us feel less hungry.

12. It's enjoyable! It has been scientifically established that after the first forty-five minutes of walking at a steady pace, the hormones endorphins are produced in the body. Endorphins, the body's natural "feel-good" hormones, are responsible for sensations of wellbeing and mental uplift. This explains why many exercisers, despite the fatigue and pain, still push themselves to their limits.

13. It is ideal for postpartum women who wish to lose weight. After months of abstaining from any physical activity during pregnancy, walking is the best way for women to lose those extra pounds.

How to walk for weight loss

Most books and websites about losing weight by walking contend that 10.000 steps a day is sufficient. Let's say you walk 10,000 steps in an hour and 10,000 steps in a whole day. Will you burn the equivalent amount in calories? *Of course not!* The 10,000 steps per day are an exceptionally effective means of boosting your health over time—but are not sufficient for you to lose weight. This amount of steps constitutes extremely good daily exercise for the heart, and is recommended by the excellent heart surgeon Magdi Yacoub, who says that he himself never goes to bed at night until the pedometer shows at least 10.000 steps!

So what is the correct way to walk if you're keen to lose weight as well benefit from the boost to your health?

To lose weight, one needs to walk at a speed of 7 to 7.5 kilometers per hour (or 7.5 to 8.5 minutes per kilometer). At this rate, the average body burns about 200 calories in half an hour.

In the personal training programs I develop, I recommend a daily 10-kilometer walk in one and a half hours. This will burn about 600 calories which, in combination with the correct diet, leads very easily and concretely to a weight loss of ½ to 1 ½ kilos weekly.

Over 1 ½ kilo per week weight loss is dangerous and definitely not going to be a permanent situation, so it is absolutely not recommended. Typically, weight loss such as this is a result of crash diets, which are often followed by a return to old eating habits as the body has been so greatly deprived. What is more, these diets are often not accompanied with the acquisition of new healthy habits such as exercise and proper and good nutrition. The result is that the weight lost is subsequently regained, with in some cases the person gaining even more than his/her original weight.

The solution is to aim for slow, steady results.

How to lose 12 kilos in 8 weeks without starving

A walking program of about 1 to 1.5 hours per day at a rate of 7.5 to 8.5 kilometers per hour, as mentioned above, will burn about 600 calories.

If this program is combined with a daily intake of 1500 calories (for the average body), this will provide a huge boost to your metabolism. It is therefore possible for someone to lose up to 1 ½ kilos of fat a week. Careful! I'm talking about 1 ½ kilos of fat! Not liquid or proteins, as is the case in most diets. And if you feel this figure is rather low, then consider that 1 ½ kilos of fat is equal to about three packets of butter (fat) of half a kilo a week! Imagine shedding three half-kilo packets of butter (fat), like that found in your refrigerator, per week! And all this with great stability and no health problems, since all you're doing is... walking. Furthermore, you will definitely not feel hungry since the 1500 calories a day is more than the usual 1200 calories recommended by most diets.

Walking also provides the ultimate in natural toning for your body during weight loss, ensuring you don't suffer from the flabby waist so common with ordinary crash diets—and what is more, as I will discuss below, you can do all this while listening to your favorite show, a seminar you've been meaning to check out, an audio book or just your favorite music!

How to start walking – program

Is it right to start at a speed of 7.5 minutes per kilometer and a distance of 10 kilometers a day? The answer depends on your personal physical condition. A person who is not a complete beginner can certainly start at this rate.

A person who is generally unfit should start cautiously. The first step is a visit to his/her doctor for a checkup. Initially, it is recommended to start walking half an hour, at a strong but steady pace.

Many people ask me what is the appropriate "strong pace." The correct answer is a pace that makes you pant and sweat—not the leisurely walking that essentially causes no tension and hence no stimulation on the cardiovascular system. This strong pace will vary according to each individual's physical condition; it will be significantly different for a marathon walker and a novice.

After fifteen days at this pace, try an hour of continuous walking at a slightly more intense pace than your initial one. Stabilize at this pace for another fifteen days. Now, after a total of 30 days of walking, the body will have begun to acclimatize; your metabolism wakes up and endorphins make their appearance. You can now start trying to pick up the speed, to reach 7.5 to 8 minutes per kilometer. Then increase the distance, to reach 8 to 10 km in total.

I would like to reiterate that the above routine is intended for a beginner, and is designed to help him/her stick to the program, by maintaining motivation and avoiding disappointment, so that he/she continues and reaches his/her goal.

In the case of a person who has some excess weight but is relatively fit, the best way to start is to measure performance. Walk for an hour at a fast pace suited to you (that makes you pant and sweat) and measure the distance walked. Repeat two more times and calculate your average speed. Then divide the time you walked (in minutes) by the distance (in kilometers). This will give you your average pace. Now, the goal is to increase this up to 7.5 to 8.0 minutes per kilometer as well as to increase the total distance you walk at 10 kilometers a day.

Trust me, you will achieve weight loss, improved health, excellent physical condition and, more importantly, you will instill good habits—essential for personal improvement and the pursuit of all our goals.

The personal improvement seminars we organize stress that an integral part of personal development is weight loss and gaining good health, not only for aesthetic reasons but also for another important reason: in personal development, everything counts!

No one who wakes up at eleven in the morning can expect everything to go smoothly at the office! No one who puts off doing difficult or laborious tasks "until tomorrow" can expect anything other than a huge backlog and a host of problems, and psychological pressure that goes with that.

No one who eats badly and is overweight expects to be full of vitality, energy and positivity, ready to perform to the max in their daily pursuit of personal goals.

"It doesn't matter if I wake up late/sleep a little longer in the morning." Wrong! Of course it matters! It harms your philosophy and your way of thinking.

"It doesn't matter if I leave the office before I've finished all today's tasks." Wrong! Of course it matters! It matters because when you leave the office you will be cogitating over the unfinished work you've left behind and you will not be able to enjoy your relaxation time at home with your family.

"It doesn't matter if I don't revise each day for my exams; I'll cram it in at the last minute and catch up." Wrong! Of course it matters! It matters because if you take this approach, you will let other courses slide and ultimately amass a huge amount of work that will be impossible to deal with and then you'll have to decide which courses you will revise, and which you will have to leave for next semester."

"It doesn't matter if I eat a cake each day—besides, it's the only joy I have left in my daily routine; it's my little escape from the trials and tribulations of my work life." Wrong! Of course it matters! It matters because your "little escape" is harming you, making you gain weight, reducing your vitality and energy levels and ultimately your productivity as well as your effectiveness at work!

Remember that all of our daily habits are inextricably linked and all together they create our attitude towards life.

In the pursuit of our personal ambitions, we need to remember that good health, a balanced mind and body, aesthetics and appearance all contribute to our personal magnetism and influence. Everything is connected—and weight loss, improved health and vitality levels will all place us firmly on the first rung of the ladder to success.

Do not expect to change your life through external factors. Change *yourself* today! If you change your daily habits, little by little each day, then over time you will change your own life too.

Start today: Improve your physical condition!

Start today: Shed that excess weight that has been tormenting you for so long!

Start walking today—for you, for your life, for your future, for your family, for your goals towards success!

START TODAY!

What is the correct way to walk?

Measure the length of a single stride. Suppose it is fifty centimeters, during normal simple walking. To calculate what it would be when walking at an intense pace, increase this length by 30% to 40%. In our example, this would be about twenty extra centimeters, giving a final length of stride of seventy centimeters. With this stride at 8 minutes per kilometer, we are on the right track.

1. Pay attention to your tread. During each step, we must ensure we use all of our tread, through the heel to the arch and ending at the toes. Although very safe, walking can cause temporary pain in the lower leg and foot tendons.

2. Maintain stable balance. It is important to keep your pelvis stable; picture balancing a glass of water on each hip. Walking works the abdominal muscles and internal organs.

3. Stand tall. Your body should be straight and stretched, with shoulders relaxed. To achieve this, pull your neck slightly upwards. This ensures your shoulders stay down and tipped slightly backwards, and is the correct posture.

4. Warm-up and cool-down. Walking, like any form of exercise, requires a warm-up at the beginning and a stretching/cool-down period at the end. A five-minute leisurely walk to start off with will prepare the body fully in terms of breathing, heart and blood circulation. At the end, give yourself five minutes during which you gradually reduce the intensity of your steps. This will drain the remnants of the lactic acid generated in the muscle cells, helping you to avoid cramps and muscle aches and pains.

Problems you may encounter

Many people taking their first steps in sports walking will feel pain in the anterior part of the tibia or in the tendon behind the ankle. This is due to the fact that when we take large, snappy strides, our feet technically act as levers, and vigorous exercise exerts pressure on these levers.

The solution for reducing or eliminating pain is firstly to wear appropriate, ergonomically designed running shoes with soft soles, and secondly to ensure you include a five-minute warm-up and five-minute cool-down. If pain persists, use one of the many anti-inflammatory preparations available at any chemist, applying it to the painful area.

How do we measure distance and pace?

There are many methods available online. These are two of my favorites:

http://www.google.com/earth/index.html

http://maps.google.gr/maps?hl=el&q=nike+%2B+running+app&bav=on.2,or.r_qf.&bvm=bv.45107431,d.ZWU&biw=1707&bih=943&wrapid=tlif136567409153510&um=1&ie=UTF-8&sa=N&tab=wl

To calculate the distance and route you're walking daily, go to Google Earth and draw the path traveled. Then calculate the total distance using the meter. Google maps works in much the same way. A handheld stopwatch or smartphone will enable you to measure the time you take to travel that distance. Once you have these measurements, you will be able to calculate your pace by dividing the distance calculated on Google Earth by the measured time—and all for zero cost.

There are a wealth of other methods out there for measuring distance, time and calories burned—even a handheld GPS (though if you don't have one already, purchasing one would be an expensive way of doing it).

A cheaper option is a pedometer—the best ones count steps, time and calories burned.

Another very good application that is free of charge, and personally I use it very often, comes from the NIKE Corporation and is intended for Android devices, smartphones, iPhones, etc.: the NIKE + Runningapp. This is an excellent application—and a cinch to install:
http://nikeplus.nike.com/plus/products/gps_app/

This application calculates your route on a map via your GPS, indicating the distance you've walked, time, and calories burned. It also has the handy feature of retaining your old times making it easy for you to compare and keep tabs on your progress. It keeps a detailed record of each separate route you've walked, and provides a sum total of all kilometers walked, as well as your personal record, such as your best time per kilometer or per mile, the longest distance per practice and much more. It even shows you which parts of your route you covered faster or slow. It has a nifty voice feature that keeps you informed of your performance and times per kilometer. And last, but certainly not least, it provides you an added incentive by rewarding virtual prizes for each significant achievement.

A similar application is the Run Keeper for your Android device. You can download it for free from the website:
http://runkeeper.com/android

This has similar characteristics to those of Nike's application. It is very reliable and gives information every 5 minutes of activity.

You should nevertheless bear in mind that the calculation of calories burned by these devices is based on simple algorithms that calculate your walking pace then multiply this by the number of calories burned per minute depending on the pace. This is the same method I described above—a calculation you can do yourself.

For example, if you walk at a speed of 8.5 min/km for 45 minutes, then, knowing that the average number of calories burned for this rate is 200 kcal/half hour means that you burn about 300 kcal in 45 minutes.

An excellent guide and one of the most accurate measurements of calories burned is provided in the table hereunder.

Table : Kcal burned in ½ hour of walking

Your weight		Kcal burned In ½ hour walking speed or pace 3.2kph 18.75min/km 2mph 30min/mile	Kcal burned in ½ hour walking speed or pace 4kph 15min/km 2.5mph 24min/mile	Kcal burned in ½ hour walking speed or pace 4.8kph 12.5min/km 3mph 20min/mile
Kg	lbs			
50	110	93	111	114
60	132	99	117	123
70	154	108	126	132
80	176	114	135	141
90	198	129	150	159
100	220	130	152	160

Your weight		Kcal burned in ½ hour walking speed or pace 5.6kph 11min/km 3.5mph 17min/km	Kcal burned in ½ hour walking speed or pace 6.4kph 9.4min/km 4mph 15min/mile	Kcal burned in ½ hour walking speed or pace 7.2kph 8min/km 4.5mph 13min/mile	Kcal burned in ½ hour walking speed or pace 8kph 7.5min/km 5mph 12min/mile
Kg	lbs				
50	110	129	165	204	240
60	132	135	177	219	258
70	154	144	189	234	276
80	176	156	201	249	294
90	198	174	225	279	327
100	220	176	227	280	330

Should you go it alone?

It's good to walk with friends if you can. If your companion has experience in long walks, that's even better because you'll have some guidance along the way and be sure to reach your correct pace without too many hiccups. Remember, though, that you should avoid talking as you walk as doing so will tire you out and probably perhaps prevent you from completing your program. At my seminars, I usually set up groups of five people and literally tag along as they walk. It's fantastic to be in good company as you walk. We generally walk about 11 kilometers early every morning.

So, start your day walking—preferably on an empty stomach, because this way the body burns more. And there is nothing better than a delicious breakfast after strenuous exercise—the perfect start to a new, creative, fantastic day.

Chapter 2: Self-Motivation

This is perhaps the most important chapter of all. So many of us make the decision at some point in our lives to slim down, to start doing some sport, to change our bodies, our mood, our lives.

Nevertheless, after a few days, most stop trying—frustrated, discouraged, sidetracked by their hectic daily routines, lack of self-discipline and willpower.

But why does this happen and what can we do to overcome it?

Think about a young child fascinated by the flame of a candle. The flame lights up people's faces, flickers and glows. The child is captivated. When he reaches out and touches the flame, however, the pain reflex makes him pull his hand back fast. He starts to associate the flame with pain. The child may try to touch the flame a few more times, but the pain is always the same, so in the end he learns not to touch it.

Exactly the same happens with people who want to change their lives. They set out along the road of change buoyed up with motivation. They start with a crash diet, swimming, running, trying to get used to the feeling of hunger. The result? Basically they experience pain and disappointment and finally, with the ongoing deprivation of food, grow moody, stressed and exhausted. Then they succumb. They start to eat larger amounts of food than they did before starting the diet, and quite happily give up whatever form of physical activity they had started.

I receive dozens of emails daily from people asking me for tips on how to stay motivated and focused on their target and, more importantly, how not to give up after trying three weeks, six weeks— even six months.

Believe me, there is nothing easier in life than to change—within a second. And it's all the *more* easy because if we really have decided to change, then nothing will prevent us from achieving what we have always dreamed of.

In the following chapters, I will describe some of the techniques you can use to achieve this.

Procrastination

How many times have you heard people saying they'll start a diet next Monday. And how many times have they then postponed it to the following Monday? Then the next—and so on, until eventually it goes on for weeks, months, years and they've made zero progress.

This small, repetitive, daily mistake means they end up with the same life they had yesterday: the same weight, same eating habits, same physical and medical problems, psychological problems—a life without glory, without beauty, without grace.

The worst counselor in pursuing any goal is that of procrastination. Procrastination is the constant postponement of starting a new effort. Postpone the decision to start eating better.
Postpone the decision to start working out regularly.
Postpone the decision to quit smoking.
Postpone the decision to complete all the pending tasks in the office before we leave left each night.
Postpone the decision to improve the way we work.
Postpone the decision to set high personal goals, which will lead us to the fulfillment of our dreams!
Everything that happens in our lives is dependent on our state of mind.
Everything you dream of—a good figure, health, beauty, love, career success, family happiness—originates as a statement, an expression and an action that starts in our mind.
Therefore, if we want to change our lives, we must change our state of mind.

Acknowledging the problem & maintaining motivation

Most people I know want to get fit, lose weight, slim down, get healthier, and improve their mood. But although they claim to want all this, they don't take any concrete action, don't do a single thing to get started or even bother to change any of their current habits. It's as if they are waiting for their life to change by magic—all on its own, or through a stranger who gives them the magic formula to succeed effortlessly and smoothly, without them having to give any of their time, thought or energy.

Wrong! Whatever it is that we seek in our lives, we have to pay the appropriate fee to conquer! We have to take the responsibility of our lives—*us*; not anybody else.

And what is it that makes them think that way?

The fear of failure!

Having tried many times in the past to change their lives—and failed—they resign themselves to the fact that it is useless to try again, just as the child realized it was useless touching the flame again and again in the hope that at some point the pain would not be there.

They fear that they will fail once again, leading to the familiar feelings of disappointment and letdown at having reneged their newfound healthier lifestyle. So they take the easy route—and postpone!

Wrong! Wrong! Wrong!

Now is the right time for you to change. **Now** is the right time to leave behind anything that is keeping you hooked on old habits. Don't expect it to happen on its own. Nothing will change suddenly of its own accord and push you into achieving what you've always wanted and dreamed of. Nothing will melt away your excess weight from one day to the next. Nothing can force you to take the decision to act—except perhaps an order from your doctor to change your lifestyle!

My goal is not to worry you, but to wake you up! To give you the little push you need to get motivated and to stay on the move!

Acknowledge the problem. We all have strong internal instincts. We know exactly what we need to do. We know exactly where we are and where we want to go. Yet when we talk with people around us, we tend to down-play or hide our problems. This is part of our body's natural defense system resulting from the instinct for self-preservation.

It's time to stop playing hide and seek with ourselves!

Record the problem. Take a sheet of paper and write down what you perceive as a problem and want to solve, to change. Write down that you want to lose weight and form new habits. That you want to improve your health, to walk for an hour four times a week; you want to start a diet of 1500 calories a day. Keep this paper carefully in a file.

Now that the problem is recorded, it becomes real. It is no longer hidden in the recesses of your mind, but declared. It exists. As such, it will niggle at you—so it must be solved.

And now is the right time to take the plunge. Since you know the problem, it must be solved! Today! Now!

Now you have to decide that you will change your life. Nor tomorrow or in a month—but now! TODAY!

The next step is to tell those around you. This is the most difficult part of the process—and you will only do this if you are truly determined to change.

Letting others know of your decision to lose weight, get fit and healthy and change your life is a means of locking yourself in to this decision.

Think about what you need in order to reach your goal. It is important to start programming your brain with new, good habits in place of the old, bad ones. Since your brain has been unconsciously programmed with poor eating habits, no exercise, no activity, collapsing on the couch as soon as you get home from work and watching TV all evening, you will need to reprogram your brain with healthier habits.

A small step at a time. One step at a time.

If you need 2500 calories a day to maintain your weight and you eat an extra biscuit every day, the extra 250 calories a day will add a whopping 12 kilos to your weight within a year (a kilogram is equivalent to about 7300 calories). Conversely, if each day you consume 250 calories less than you need, respectively, in one year you will have lost 12 kilos! Without doing anything else at all!

It becomes readily apparent that success is as far from failure as a biscuit!

So, **number one is our internal decision.**

Changing small habits today will have a great impact on our lives tomorrow. Put an end to procrastination! We only have one life! By postponing things to "another day," we just end up spending our entire lives waiting for something to change!

You are the protagonist. Stop admiring others for their achievements and take responsibility for *your* life in *your* hands today.

You are a unique person. You deserve it and you will get it.

Make this promise to yourself.

Read through the useful tips in the following chapters and keep on moving through. Do not look back.

Half of the journey to success is taking the decision!

So take that decision now!

Self-Discipline

Another important factor to ensure you stay motivated and stick to your healthier lifestyle is self-discipline. Even if you take that initial decision to get fit, unless you stick religiously to the program you have set yourself, you will never succeed.

The secret is to trick your mind into sticking to the plan. I know many businesspeople who work extremely hard from early morning until late at night and claim that it is impossible to find time to exercise—and perhaps this is the case. But there are plenty of examples to the contrary.

Take Neil Bates, for example, who works in an IT company in London. As is the case for so many people who say they don't have the time to exercise, his daily schedule was hectic. We first met at a seminar in Crete and when he explained his daily routine to me, I truly felt he was the absolute personification of a workaholic. His eating habits were dreadful—fast food at the office; his physical activity was practically zero; his medical indicators had hit red and his doctors had warned him of the very serious health risks he was running. According to him, however, it was impossible to change anything in his daily schedule.

We talked several hours and finally arrived at the following simple solution.

First: he would leave his car at home.

Second: Each morning he would go to work on foot. He would get off the tube three stations before his usual stop and walk the three kilometers to his office. He would do the same on the way home.

Third: He would take the stairs whenever there were any—to the subway, at the office and elsewhere.

Fourth: He would at a balanced, 1500-calorie diet.

These four basic steps did not change anything major in his daily schedule.

Within four months, he had lost 20 kilos! He felt healthy, strong, had acquired good eating habits and now declares that he has changed his life. Today, he walks 10 km in 1.5 hours three times a week (two of which are on Saturday and Sunday when he has more time). We speak regularly and I am sincerely happy about the improvements he has made to his life and health.

Next, Jim O'Ralley. Jim lives in Vancouver, and sent me an email explaining that he found it hard to stick to his walking program because he got distracted and he'd now dropped his pace. He'd tried to motivate himself by listening to music as he walked, but it didn't work. Jim was facing exactly what the vast majority of people face when they attempt to introduce physical activity into their lives: lack of concentration and staying power.

Jim works as a mechanical engineer with a mining company. In one our discussions he told me he just didn't have any spare time: he worked 12-hour days, seven days a week and hardly even saw his family. He never had any time to himself and had recently started a master's degree program, which made it even more difficult for him to fit his walking program in. He had tried for 20 days to stay loyal to the program, but was growing less and less motivated.

After our chat, I suggested that he record the lessons for his master's degree on an MP3 player, or get audio books from the university, so that he could listen to them as he walked. This would save him precious time.

This move proved highly successful. Within one year, Jim had completed his master's and lost 40 kilos thanks to lengthy walks and good nutrition.

Essentially, what he did was shift his mindset so that he thought about his walking as an integral part of his daily studying for his master's degree—which was something he was highly motivated to achieve.

So, he studied as he walked—and lost weight as he studied!

Isn't it amazing?

George Georgopoulos worked on the 43rd floor of the Empire Estate. A few years ago, he was a hard-working businessman who always had an excuse not to work out. After much thought and deliberation, he decided to leave the car at home and start a walking program—which had truly impressive results.

Today, George walks daily for one hour. Most impressive, though, is that he climbs up and down the stairs to his office at least twice a day, 43 floors up! Now, *that's* willpower. He has a busy schedule, like many other people, but he's doing a great job. He's lost 22 kilos and his health is excellent, as is his physical appearance.

Anna Kearns had a difficult pregnancy, during which she gained more than 22 kilos. The labor was complicated and when she finally returned to a normal daily rhythm, she realized how difficult it was to shift the twelve kilos she'd put on.

She struggled for hours in gyms lifting weights or running in the hallways. But her eating habits had changed significantly, especially since she was comfort eating as a result of new pressures at her place of work. A new employee had taken over her position during her maternity leave at the advertising company she worked for and now she had to prove not only that she was capable of returning after several months' maternity leave, but also that she was more capable than her new competitor! She felt insignificant, unattractive and overweight.

We met at a seminar in Athens. She combined attending the seminar with a vacation in the Greek Islands. We started a daily walking program for about an hour along the shore, and introduced a carefully developed diet containing specific foods that help you feel full and satiated quickly. We were together at the seminar for a month. The day she flew back to London she had lost 8 kilos! But the most important thing is that today, three years on, she still walks every day, sticks to a healthy diet—and of course she has now lost all the pregnancy weight she had gained...

There are countless stories like these, of individuals who have taken a decision to change their lives. People with full daily schedules, almost no free time and high levels of stress—yet they do make it. There is nothing an individual cannot achieve; you just need to make up your mind, start to put in the effort and be disciplined!

Mindset is the key: things are only as easy or as difficult as we allow them to be.

Read books, attend seminars, get support

When it comes to getting fit, people often set out with the best intentions, only to give up further down the line, unable to stick to their healthier diet and physical exercise regime. Don't quit. There's a wealth of tricks and ideas to help you stick to it.

Some of the best ways to motivate you to stick to your new lifestyle are to buy books, audio books, attend seminars and find mentors who will monitor your progress daily and, most importantly, keep tabs on your frame of mind, keeping you on track to ensure you attain your goal.

During my seminars in recent years, I have seen the power of being mentored. There is a critical point we all reach when the right support from the right people can make the difference between success and failure.

During our seminars we cover personal as well as professional development, financial implications, improvements to health, and weight loss. Over the years, I have found that the fundamental requirement for achieving success is to take care of the temple of our soul—our body. My experience has shown me time and again that, for millions of people, weight problems are related to poor health.

We thing established a team of psychologists, dietitians and trainers who provide ancillary support and mentoring to busy people who feel that they need guidance and psychological support along their journey to better health and fitness.

There are many websites, mentors and experts in this field. Do not hesitate to ask for help if you see that your efforts are not paying off. There is nothing wrong with asking for help and accepting that you can not do it by yourself when you feel that you have exhausted every avenue. What *would* be wrong would be giving up without asking for help.

Holidays and changing your mindset

For many people, a holiday means good food, total relaxation, sea and sun! All of this in moderation is great. But a holiday can also mean something else: a brilliant opportunity to start changing your lifestyle.

Wake up early in the morning and walk with intensity for 1.5 hours. Then swim. Try a delicious breakfast of oranges, mango, cucumber and yogurt or two slices of wholegrain bread with honey. Enjoy the sea and sun, lose weight and get fit.

I come from Greece and I know how easy and pleasurable it is to begin your walking schedule when you're on vacation. There is no better time to embark on this journey: enjoying your vacation, losing weight, meeting people and of course swimming at the beach or in the pool.

With the global economic crisis of the past years, people are tending to eat more and more badly. Physical activity is almost nonexistent for many, and physical condition goes downhill.

But we all go on holiday. If you seize this opportunity and use it wisely, you will be a winner.

Take the stairs

Walking up and down stairs is an excellent form of exercise. It burns calories, stimulates the metabolism and prepares the body for walking.

People who start walking and nutrition programs commonly stop using the elevator and opt for the stairs instead.

Believe me, it's very easy. Once you make this small change in your life, you will not want to stop.

One could even use the argument that it is politically correct—since it reduces your carbon footprint in terms of energy consumption. Just think how much the planet would benefit if everyone were to cut down their energy consumption.

Chapter 3: Is just walking enough?

Of course not! No single physical activity is sufficient to lose weight. Suppose you're working out five hours every day, burning 2000 calories and you consume 5000 calories a day. When you're not working out, your lifestyle is pretty sedentary, so your daily nutritional requirements will be at around 4000 calories. Since you are consuming 5000 calories a day, you are consuming 1000 calories more than your daily requirements. This additional 1000 calories a day will—you guessed it—turn into fat! That means that within a month you will have a caloric surplus of 1000 calories x 30 days = 30.000 calories, which means approximately 4 kg per month or 48 kilos a year! And all this for someone who works out five hours a day!

As you can see, in this scenario you will gain weight rather than lose it, despite five hours of daily activity. This demonstrates very clearly that physical activity alone is not enough—and the same goes for diet.

You need both activity *and* proper nutrition. Scientific studies have shown that, statistically, 80% of people who lose a lot of weight by just dieting will return over time to their original weight—whereas the percentage for people who combine physical activity and proper activity is only 15%! So only 15% of people who lose weight through a combination of physical activity and proper nutrition will return to their pre-program weight over time!

This small percentage is due to the fact that physical activity tends to create a sense of satiety, meaning that you will feel less hungry less and therefore eat less. Physical activity also helps you burn off those extra calories you may have consumed when giving in to the temptation of a dessert or snack.

In conclusion, we must bear in mind that the strongest combination is WALKING and CORRECT NUTRITION.

What is the best diet?

This is the most common question asked by people who are troubled with excess weight and trying to find the best diet plan to help them shift it. Since we have already concluded that walking should be combined with proper diet, let's take a look at what is ultimately the right diet, the proper diet.

A quick search on Google will come up with thousands of different diets: 600-calorie diets, juice diets, Atkins, Dukan, vegetarian, pineapple, liquid—there are literally thousands. There is a joke about a seafood diet: "I'm on a seafood diet. Every time I see food, I eat it!"

But what is ultimately the best diet? In order to function properly, the human body needs specific nutrients. What are these?

Proteins
Proteins are essential for growth and cell renewal. We find them mostly in foods such as meat, fish, milk, eggs and legumes. They should constitute 20 to 25% of total daily calorie intake.

Fat
Fats are essential to the body because they provide energy, supplying the body with essential fatty acids and facilitating the absorption of certain vitamins. We fine fats in whole-milk products, meat, fish, nuts, olive oil and vegetable oils. Fats must not exceed 35% of total daily calorie intake, and animal fats should be less than 10% total daily calorie intake.

Carbohydrates
Carbohydrates are essential for the body to function. They provide instant energy to our body and help with the proper functioning of the brain. They are found in sugars and starches such as fruits, vegetables, honey, milk, sugar, bread, potatoes, rice, cereals. Note that more than half the calories you consume per day should come mainly from starchy carbohydrates.

Fiber
Very important for proper bowel function. We find fiber in black bread, cereals, legumes, fruits, vegetables. Fiber should constitute 3% - 4% of total daily calorie intake.

How to lose weight

The human body needs all of the above nutrients on a daily basis. For this reason, extreme diets that restrict any of these categories should not be followed as they deprive the body of nutrients that are essential for our body's proper functioning.

How is weight loss achieved?

WEIGHT LOSS
occurs when the energy you expend during daily activity and exercise is greater than the energy you obtain from food.
WEIGHT GAIN
occurs when the energy you obtain from food is greater than the energy you expend during daily activity and exercise.
Therefore, **Weight Loss is achieved by:** - Using up energy during physical activity - Reducing daily calorie intake

There is no magic, rocket science or miracle. It is a simple balance. If a person manages to control and regulate this on a daily basis, then he/she will achieve the desired result:

WEIGHT LOSS + HEALTH + FITNESS

Water: drink fearlessly

Our body is composed of 70% water and other liquids. Water is a natural lubricant that ensures the smooth running of the chemical processes taking place inside our bodies.

Scientific research in many universities has shown that water plays an important regulatory role in the slimming process.

Research suggests that 8 to 10 glasses of water a day help significantly with dieting, as a well-hydrated body will function correctly, ensuring the correct functioning of all the chemical molecules.

Also, water improves our skin quality, contributing to a more youthful appearance.

Avoid packaged foods and preservatives

Preservatives are used widely these days in processed and packaged foods, conserving them as they are transported from the source to the supermarket shelves, where they then sit until purchased by the consumer. Unfortunately, preservatives are generally toxic to the human body. They generate free radicals resulting in rapid aging and death of cells. The choice is yours: healthy and long-living cells or not!

Anger - Stress - Anxiety

The trials and tribulations of modern-day life, coupled with uncertainty about the future cause stress and anxiety for many of us today.

It is statistically proven that during times of great stress, people consume larger amounts of food and junk food. It makes sense, therefore, to be able to control our stress.

One good tactic is to never sit down at the table when you are under a high level of pressure and stress. Listen to some relaxing music, go for a walk around the block, try to think of pleasant things, or do a little meditation. Trust me—it works superbly.

Prepare your own snacks

A major challenge people face during any weight loss program is that feeling of hunger that can strike at any time of the day (or night), when you feel that if you don't eat something right away you might collapse— and you end up consuming the first snack you can get your hands on. This is one of the most fattening and bad habits.

You are not going to collapse. What happens is that when you still have several hours to go before your next meal, you can feel anxious; this triggers the production of acids in your stomach, which cause this unpleasant sensation. At this point, people often crack and eat high-calorie snacks such as pies, donuts and cookies, which obviously destroys all the great results you have achieved so far.

What should I do? Prepare healthy snacks that you will have on hand when these moments occur. Fill a large salad bowl with cabbage, carrot, lettuce, tomato, peppers and put it in the fridge for when you need it. Careful—salads must be prepared without any fattening sauce or dressing; a little lemon or vinegar and a pinch of salt makes a healthy alternative. Take sweet red apples, a banana or orange to work with you—these are great snacks for re-energizing your body.

Eat your food slowly

It takes about 20 minutes for the stomach to signal to the brain that it is full. So when you eat fast, your stomach will be full way before your brain has received the message. This means that you will eat more than you need and end up with a bloated stomach, malaise and asthenia.

Breakfast

Don't ever skip breakfast. During the night, your body fasts for a lengthy period. When you wake in the morning you need immediate energy to start your day—and breakfast does just that: breaks the fast. If you leave home without breakfast, your body will take the energy it needs directly from your energy reserves, such as stored carbohydrates or protein, rather than from your fat reserves. This will result in fatigue, weakness, loss of concentration, stomach disorders—obviously not ideal for setting you up to cope with a busy day in the workplace.

Eat foods that satiate but don't cause weight gain

Certain foods are more satiating than others. Such foods are, for example, those containing carbohydrates, such as potatoes. According to research, boiled potatoes fill us up us twice as much as chips. In contrast, fatty foods make us eat more. Highly satiating foods include boiled potatoes, oranges, fish, apples, grapes and wholegrain bread.

On the other hand, cakes, donuts and croissants are very low-satiating foods.

So choose foods with a high level of satiety—they will satisfy you and fill you up.

Watch out for alcohol and candy

There's an old saying that says that men get fat on alcohol and women on candy!

It's very true. Alcohol and candy are packed with calories but no nutrients and ultimately make us fat without us even realizing it's happening. In addition, candy and alcohol increase the feeling of hunger, often leading to a massive calorie intake overload.

A glass of red wine with your meal is a sensible option; indeed, research shows that a glass of red wine from time to time can actually have positive health benefits.

A dessert of ice cream and fruits is also a good choice.

Keep a record of what you eat

Keep a journal of what you eat and whether you've stuck to or deviated from your program. It is important to monitor, at least in the beginning, exactly what you eat and how many times—if any—you strayed from the program.

Many people grow frustrated when they deviate from their program one, two, three or more times, and end up giving up altogether If you keep a record of what you've eaten, you will be able to monitor your intake and take corrective action to ensure you stay on track.

For example, if you have eaten 1000 extra calories one week, then by just eating 200 calories less each day for the next 10 days, you will be in equilibrium; or by walking half an hour more for three days a week, within 1.5 weeks you'll be back on track in your original program.

Calculate how many calories you need to stay at your current weight. Then decide how much walking you need to do and how many calories you need to consume per day in order to gradually and steadily lose weight.

———————————————

Chapter 4: How Many Calories Do We Need?

Calculating your basal metabolic rate

First you need to calculate your basal metabolic rate; i.e., the number of calories you need to consume daily in order to maintain a stable weight and carry out normal everyday activities.

Below I list two of the clearest, most reliable methods for calculating basal metabolic rate. These methods were developed based on long-term studies on a large number of people.

Method 1

AGE	CALORIES PER DAY
15 - 18 years	(17.6 x W) + 656
18 - 30 years	(15 x W) + 690
30 – 60 years	(11.4 x W) + 870
Over 60 years	(11.7 x W) + 585

Weight in kilos

Example:
If you are a woman aged 32 and weigh 62 kilos, your basal metabolic (BM) rate is calculated as follows:

BM = 11.4 x 62 + 690 $\Rightarrow$ BM = 888 + 485 = 1.397 kcal.

Note that the height is not taken into account at all in this method.

Method 2

This method is considered by most nutritionists to be the most reliable and accurate as it takes height into consideration.

Women : BM = 655 + (9.6 x W) + (1.8 x H) - (4.7 x A)
Men   : BM = 66 + (13.7 x W) + (5 x H) - (6.8 x A)

BM = Basal metabolic rate
W = W in kilos
H = Height in cm
A = Age in years

Example:
Let's suppose that the woman in the previous example is 170 cm tall. The calculation would be as follows:

BM = 655 + (9.6 x 62) + (1.8 x 170) - (4.7 x 32)
BM = 655 + 595 + 306 - 150 = 1.406 kcal.

As you will see, the end result obtained using each method is very close.

Note: Since people are all different, these equations, which are based on studies involving a large number of people, will never be identical and will always show a slight discrepancy in the number of calories. This is why scientists, nutritionists, biochemists and others have not been able to develop a unique common way of calculating basal metabolic rate.

Measuring your daily natural energy expenditure

Once you have calculated your basal metabolic rate, the next step is to find the energy you expend each day through physical activity. To calculate this, you first need to record all of your activities during a 24-hour period. Each activity has a corresponding rate, as shown in the table hereunder.

Next, you need to calculate the average rate, which when multiplied by the basal metabolic rate gives us the energy we expend within a day.

Note: The various estimates of caloric needs-based equations should be regarded as indicative rather than absolute, since energy needs vary from individual to individual and from day to day, hour to hour and second to second. Even the smallest physical movement uses up energy, which is difficult to calculate accurately.

Categories of activities and intensity factor for each

Categories of activities	Intensity factor
Rest and Sleep	1.0
Very light work - exercise Activities in a sitting or standing position, typewriting, sewing, ironing, cooking, playing musical instrument, laboratory work	1.5
Light work - exercise Simple walking on a flat surface/street at 4-5 km per hour, working in a restaurant, housework, woodwork, childcare, working in the garage, sailing	2.5
Moderate work - exercise Fast walking 5.5 - 6.5 km per hour, carrying heavy loads, dancing, skiing, cycling, tennis, digging	5.0
Heavy work - very fast walking 7.5 - 8 km per hour, basketball, soccer, digging, climbing	7.0

Source: World Health Organization, 2005.

Example:

If you slept for eight hours, worked at your office and later at home on your computer for a total of 10 hours, then played with your children or worked in the garage (light work) for 4 hours and then walked vigorously (heavy work) for 2 hours, then multiply the hours spent in each activity category by the corresponding intensity factor of the activity, as follows:

- Hours of rest x 1.0 = [8]
- 10 hours very light work x 1.5 = [15]
- 4 hours light work x 2.5 = [10]
- 2 hours heavy work x 7.0 = [14]

Now sum up the results: [8 + 15 + 10 + 14 = 47]

Then divide the total sum (i.e., 47) by 24 (hours in a full day):
47: 24 = 1.9.

The result of this operation (i.e., 1.9) represents the average rate of physical activity for the day in question.

To find the total energy expended through your basal metabolic rate and physical activity, multiply the calories for your basal metabolic rate by the average rate of physical activity.

Number of calories needed to maintain energy balance and weight	=	Basal Metabolic Rate (Calories)	x	Average activity factor

Thus, in accordance with the example above, the total energy consumed for that specific day is:

Total Energy = Basal Metabolic Rate x Average Activity Factor
= 1397 Kcal x 1.9 = 3,893

The resulting number is the quantity of calories you should consume daily to maintain your weight. Any calorie consumption below this figure obviously leads to weight loss!

If, on doing this calculation, you see that your physical activity index is less than 1.75, then your risk of obesity is considerable. A physical activity index of more than 1.8 means you are at a very high risk of obesity.

How many calories should I eat to maintain or lose weight?

To maintain your weight, your daily calorie intake should not exceed the number of calories indicated in your total energy expenditure calculation.

Now, if you want to slim down, you must either reduce your daily calorie intake through diet, or burn more calories—always by walking!

The best option would be a combination of both. Since a kilo (2.2 lbs) of fat contains about 7300 calories, a daily reduction of 500 calories in your diet means that by the end of the week you will have lost about half a pound of fat.

Therefore, in order to achieve a steady weight loss of about 1 to 1.5 kilos per week (4-6 kilos a month), you should consume about 1000 to 1500 calories less than your current daily consumption (in the previous example: 3893 - 1500 = 2393 calories).

According to experts, weight loss of 1 to 1.5 pounds a week is safe for your health. But beware; don't be seduced by diets that promise quick weight loss, based on less than 1200 calories a day, because not only will this deprive you of vitamins and minerals that are essential for your body, but this will slow down your metabolism, making weight loss even harder and putting your health at risk.

Below are some excellent, proven diet plans for daily calorie intakes of 1200, 1600 or 1800 calories. Please note that these menus are just suggestions; there are a multitude of menus available that you can use for effective weight loss in combination with your walking program.

1200-Calorie Daily Diet

BREAKFAST
Milk 1 cup (250 ml) 0% fat
1 slice of bread (30 g.)
or
1 slice of bread (45 g.)
5 large or 10 small olives
Decoction unsweetened

Brunch 10 am
1 fruit 120 g. (apple, orange, pear, 3 apricots, 12 large cherries, 1 peach, 8 loquat, quince 300g., pomegranate 200 g.)

LUNCH
Meal 1:
1 slice of bread (30 g.) 100 g. meat (cooked) or 100 g. chicken (cooked) or 150 g. fish (cooked) and green salad with 2 teaspoons oil.

Meal 2:
1 slice of bread (30 g.), 1 cup cooked lentils and salad (moderate tomato 1) with 4 teaspoons oil.

Afternoon 5:00 p.m.
1 fruit

DINNER
Meal 1:
1 slice of bread (30 g.), 1 cup cooked lentils and salad (moderate tomato 1) with 4 teaspoons oil.

Meal 2:
1 slice of bread (30 g.) 100 g. meat (cooked) or 100 g. chicken (cooked) or 150 g. fish (cooked) and green salad with 2 teaspoons oil.

Before bedtime
1 fruit

1600-Calorie Daily Diet

BREAKFAST
Milk 1 cup (250 ml) 0% or 3% fat
2 slices bread (60 g.)
or
2 slices bread (60 g.)
5 large or 10 small olives
Decoction unsweetened

Brunch 10 am
1 fruit 120 g. (apple, orange, pear, 3 apricots, 12 large cherries, 1 peach, 8 loquat, quince 300g., pomegranate 200 g.)

LUNCH
Meal 1:
1 slice of bread (30 g.) and 1 cup cooked lentils and salad (moderate tomato 1) 5 teaspoons oil.

Meal 2:
2 slices of bread (60 g) and 100 g. meat (cooked) and green salad with 2 tablespoons oil and half fruit.

Afternoon 5:00 p.m.
1 fruit

DINNER
Meal 1:
2 slices of bread (60 g) and 100 g. meat (cooked) and green salad with 2 tablespoons oil and half fruit.

Meal 2:
1 slice of bread (30 g.) and 1 cup lentils or peas (cooked) and salad (moderate tomato 1) 5 teaspoons oil.

Before bedtime
1 fruit 120 g.

1800-Calorie Daily Diet

BREAKFAST
Milk 1 cup (250 ml) 0% or 3% fat
2 slices bread (60 g.)
or
2 slices bread (60 g.)
10 large or 20 small olives
Decoction unsweetened

Brunch 10 am
1 slice of bread and 30 g. cheese

LUNCH
Meal 1:
1 slice of bread (30 g.) and 1 cup cooked lentils and salad (moderate tomato 1) with 5 teaspoons of oil and 1 fruit.

Meal 2:
2 slices of bread (60 g) and 100 g. meat (cooked) or 120 g. chicken (cooked) or 150 g. fish (cooked) and salad (1 medium tomato) with 3 teaspoons oil and 1 fruit.

Afternoon 5.00 p.m.
1 fruit

DINNER
Meal 1:
2 slices of bread (60 g) and 100 g. meat (cooked) or 120 g. chicken (cooked) or 150 g. fish (cooked) and salad (1 medium tomato) with 3 teaspoons oil and 1 fruit.

Meal 2:
1 slice of bread (30 g.) and 1 cup cooked lentils and peas or salad (1 medium tomato) with 5 teaspoons of oil and 1 fruit.

Before bedtime
1 fruit 120 g. 1 small or yogurt (250 g. 2% fat) milk or 1 cup (250 g. 2% fat).

Food Substitutes

FRUIT
1 apple 120g can be replaced with:
1 medium pear
1 medium peach
2 medium apricots
8 loquats
1 kiwi
½ grapefruit 300 g.
1 slice of watermelon
1 large tangerine
10 large cherries
½ banana
1 pomegranate 220 g.
1 nectarine
Three plums
1 slice of melon 250 g.
1 medium orange
1 cup strawberries
Quince 300 g.
Pineapple 150 g.

Breads, cereals, legumes and starchy vegetables
1 thin slice of bread 30 g. (80 kcal) can be replaced with:
1 slice bran bread (35 g.)
1 slice rye bread (35 g.)
2.5 crackers (20 g.)
2 small toasts
½ cup cornflakes (20 g.)
½ cup rice, pasta
2 tsp. rice, pasta, wheat
½ cup spaghetti noodles

½ cup beans, chickpeas, lentils
Beans, chickpeas, lentils
1 small potato (100 g.)
½ cup purée
½ cup zucchini (100 g.)
⅓ cup wheat, corn (80 g.)
1 small baked corn (100 g.)

MEAT, CHICKEN, FISH, CHEESE
100 g. cooked lean beef can be replaced by the same quantity of:
Beef
Mince
Pork
Chicken
Skinless turkey
Low-fat cheese.

FATS
1 teaspoon olive oil (45 kcal) can be replaced with:
1 tsp. sweet margarine
1 tsp. sweet butter
1 tsp. sweet mayonnaise
1 tsp. sweet cream cheese
5 large or 10 small olives
1 tsp. of sour cream
1 slice of bacon
20 microns peanuts
6 small nuts
5 microns almonds

MILK
Whole milk 1 cup (150 kcal) can be replaced with:
½ cup evaporated milk
1 whole-milk yogurt
cup of skim milk (90 kcal) can be replaced with:
½ cup evaporated skim milk
½ cup skim milk powder
1 yogurt from skim milk (0-2%)

INDICATIVE PROGRAM FOR BEGINNERS

FIRST 15 DAYS

DAY	ROUTINE
MONDAY	20 MINUTES BRISK WALKING
	5 MINUTES EASY WALKING
	20 ΛΕΠΤΑ BRISK WALKING
	5 MINUTES EASY WALKING
TUESDAY	DAY OFF
WEDNESDAY	20 MINUTES BRISK WALKING
	5 MINUTES EASY WALKING
	20 ΛΕΠΤΑ BRISK WALKING
	5 MINUTES EASY WALKING
THURSDAY	DAY OFF
FRIDAY	20 MINUTES BRISK WALKING
	5 MINUTES EASY WALKING
	20 MINUTES BRISK WALKING
	5 MINUTES EASY WALKING
SATURDAY	20 MINUTES BRISK WALKING
	5 MINUTES EASY WALKING
	20 MINUTES BRISK WALKING
	5 MINUTES EASY WALKING
SUNDAY	20 MINUTES BRISK WALKING
	5 MINUTES EASY WALKING
	20 MINUTES BRISK WALKING
	5 MINUTES EASY WALKING

INDICATIVE PROGRAM FOR BEGINNERS

NEXT 15 DAYS

DAY	ROUTINE
	40 MINUTES WALKING PACE 8.5min/km
MONDAY	15 MINUTES EASY WALKING
TUESDAY	DAY OFF
WEDNESDAY	40 MINUTES WALKING PACE 8.5min/km
	15 MINUTES EASY WALKING
THURSDAY	DAY OFF
FRIDAY	40 MINUTES WALKING PACE 8.5min/km
	15 MINUTES EASY WALKING
SATURDAY	40 MINUTES WALKING PACE 8.5min/km
	15 MINUTES EASY WALKING
SUNDAY	40 MINUTES WALKING PACE 8.5min/km
	15 MINUTES EASY WALKING

INDICATIVE PROGRAMME FOR ADVANCED

DAY	ROUTINE
MONDAY	60 MINUTES WALKING PACE 7.5min/km
TUESDAY	60 MINUTES WALKING PACE 7.5min/km
WEDNESDAY	60 MINUTES WALKING PACE 7.5min/km
THURSDAY	DAY OFF
FRIDAY	60 MINUTES WALKING PACE 7.5min/km
SATURDAY	60 MINUTES WALKING PACE 7.5min/km
SUNDAY	60 MINUTES WALKING PACE 7.5min/km

INDICATIVE PROGRAMME FOR ADVANCED

DAY	ROUTINE
MONDAY	60 MINUTES WALKING PACE 7min/km
TUESDAY	75 MINUTES WALKING PACE 7min/km
WEDNESDAY	60 MINUTES WALKING PACE 7min/km
THURSDAY	DAY OFF
FRIDAY	75 MINUTES WALKING PACE 7min/km
SATURDAY	60 MINUTES WALKING PACE 7min/km
SUNDAY	75 MINUTES WALKING PACE 7min/km

Tips

- Walk as much as you can. You'll burn fat and improve your health.
- Leave your car at home.
- Walk to work. It's good for your health, your pocket and the environment.
- Get off the bus or tube one or two stations before your usual stop and walk. Do the same going home.
- Climb stairs at home, at the office, your clients' offices, at the store. Don't use the elevator.
- Make MP3 recordings of topics of interest to you and listen to them as you walk. You will be focused on your audio and won't even realize you're exercising—ideal for walking.
- It is best to avoid listening to music because it creates emotional feelings and associations that do not help in walking.
- Keep track of your performance. It is important to know when, where and how much you walked. This way you can keep track of your progress.
- When you start, keep a record of the calories you consume for a week so you know your exact calorie intake and its source.
- Read books about walking. Watch seminars and talk to experts who will support and help you to develop your schedule.
- Decide that you want to lose weight and become healthier. Record your decision. Declare to everybody that from this moment on, you will be changing your life. Now you can't go back on your word!
- Drink plenty of water—it's a fabulous weight loss aid.
- Find some friends who are willing to commit to walking with you. It's great to have company, especially in the early days.
- Do not expect instant results. Give yourself a time limit of one month, walk and eat a sensible diet. If after one month you don't start to feel better about yourself, change sport!
- Reduce your daily calorie intake. Eat plenty of highly satiating foods that fill you up and cut hunger.
- Share your results with others. It will help you stay on target.
- Download apps such as "NIKE app+" and have fun with your performance and new records.
- Do not rush to see the results. Do not measure your weight daily and do not monitor the changes to your body shape. Allow the first month of walking to pass by and then you will definitely see the changes more

intensely.
• Include 2 to 3 tablespoons of extra virgin olive oil in your daily diet—Greek, Italian or Spanish are excellent varieties.
• Maintain good posture, keeping your upper body erect. This will work your abdominal muscles and tone up your abdomen.

And Finally...

Thousands of people have changed their lifestyles through walking. It is proven that walking will help you lose weight, get fit and improve your health—all of which will contribute toward helping you achieve your life goals.

Your body is the temple of your soul. The better you treat it, the more it will reward you. It goes something like this: Make an investment and you will be rewarded. If you invest nothing, you will get nothing. If you invest a few hours a week in your walking, you will be rewarded with good health, a slim body and vitality, putting you in good stead to successful achieve all of your life goals.

Change your life now!

Why not—and why not now?

God bless you all and... keep walking!

About the Author

Andy Bakas is an author, entrepreneur and personal development trainer.
He has two bachelor's degrees and a master's degree and has trained many people to achieve their goals.

He is the founder of the Master Walking Club.

He believes that nothing is impossible as long as you are keen to succeed!

For contact : email. andy_bakas@yahoo.com

_____

Printed in Great Britain
by Amazon